THE RAW GREEK

Natural,nutritious alternatives to Greek cuisine
made from 100% raw ingredients

GINA PANAYI

Note for Librarians: A cataloguing record for this book is available from Library and
Archives Canada at www.collectionscanada.ca/amicus/index-e.html
ISBN 1-4120-9340-6

Writing and Photography
Gina Panayi
gina@therawgreek.com - www.therawgreek.com

Front Cover Design
Simply White Design

Printing
Vibrant Print and Design Ltd
www.vibrantprint.com

Offices in Canada, USA, Ireland and UK

Book sales for North America and international:
Trafford Publishing, 6E–2333 Government St.,
Victoria, BC aV8T 4P4 CANADA
phone 250 383 6864 (toll-free 1 888 232 4444)
fax 250 383 6804; email to orders@trafford.com
Book sales in Europe:
Trafford Publishing (Q<) Limited, 9 Park End Street, 2nd Floor
Oxford, UK OX1 1HH UNITED KINGDOM
phone 44 (0)1865 722 113 (local rate 0845 230 9601)
facsimile 44 (0)1865 722 868; info.uk@trafford.com
Order online at:
trafford.com/06-1094
10 9 8 7 6 5 4 3 2 1

DEDICATION

To Mum and Dad. Thank you for giving me life, nurturing my needs and being patient and understanding during my personal evolution.

I love you both with all my heart; you have made me who I am today.

ACKNOWLEDGMENTS

Chad Sarno. You took me into your kitchen and inspired me.

Daniel Vitalis. For showing me the right path and being passionate about everything you believe in, we should all live by your example.

Natalie Cole. You truly are a great friend and I am forever grateful for all your help with this book and all my raw food endeavors, every chef needs a Nat in their kitchen to clean up, even if they haven't finished with the knife and chopping board yet. I admire your patience and drive.

Mum. You've tried every single dish in this book and guided me through the wonderful flavours of Greek cuisine. You've sacrificed your kitchen on many occasions and even suffered with washing up, I could not have done this without you.

Rena. For saving the day

Katy. For lifting the tone

To everyone else who is in my life, without the support, laughter, tears, advice and love I would not be where I am today, I can't thank you enough.

"Vitality and beauty are gifts from nature for those who live according to its laws."

Leonardo DaVinci

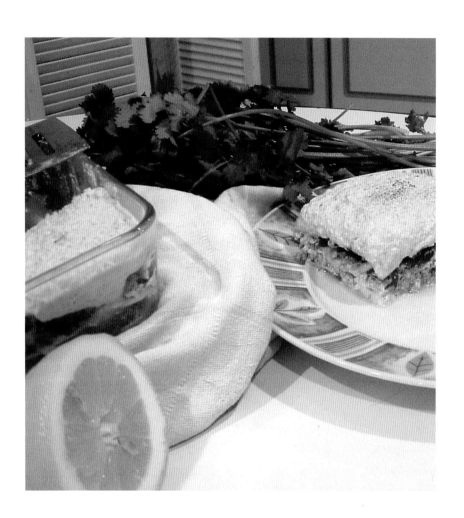

CONTENTS

Foreword by Chad Sarno

"Within the vegan and raw culinary world you will find a very broad range of chefs, from the few restaurant experienced to home grown self taught, to recipe developers. One of the rarities to come by within this growing, vast field and within raw preparation books on the market is true cultural cuisine that magnifies traditional flavors. Gina has taken this step to bring the authenticity back to the raw table, merging traditional flavors of her cultural background to the present light of raw food preparation. Having the opportunity to have Gina in a number of my kitchens for events has been a pleasure and has revealed her natural, passionate and simple approach to what she emanates the most; bringing the importance of this potent lifestyle to the masses. This book is a wonderful tool to do so and I am sure you will agree once you've had a read."

Have you...

...ever stopped to wonder why all diets, healthy eating regimes, anti aging and anti carcinogenic (cancerous) cures begin with fresh, raw, organic fruit and vegetables? Any sensible diet will tell you to snack on fruit throughout the day instead of sugary processed foods and to include more fresh vegetables when preparing meals. A handful of raw nuts or seeds are commonly suggested as an alternative to the salted variety or a packet of crisps. With so much good advice you may wonder why there are still so many people with major health issues.

There have been well known disputes amongst doctors as to what the 'right' diet is. Some say that vegetarian diets do not have sufficient protein, others that a high protein diet is dangerous and can cause high cholesterol. There are so many conflicting opinions coming from the medical community that I believe it is about time we started thinking for ourselves.

Different opinions expressed by the weight loss industry about how we should live present an immense threat to society, encouraging us to constantly look at eating habits as a diet by which to lose weight, as opposed to a healthy eating regime or lifestyle. It should not all be about what tastes good but also about how it makes you feel and how your body reacts internally as well as externally. Changes in our eating and drinking habits can lead to changes in our health. What we eat not only affects our day-to-day health but also helps to determine our quality of life and how long we live.

Fruit and Vegetables are reported to contain anti cancerous nutrients that can help the human body fight against one of the biggest threats we are facing in human life today. Fruit and vegetables are also known to slow down the fast aging process that today's polluted lifestyle can cause.

Convenience foods are tempting our minds against what we know is the right way to eat to help us feel physically better and mentally stronger. Often those that are striving towards healthier living are attacked and constantly challenged about their 'strange eating habits', myself included, when I shocked my meat eating Greek family by becoming vegetarian and consequently vegan. Well, I have news for you! It is the fast food consumer, who has been easily led into adopting an inhumane eating lifestyle.

2

We all know about the short energy boosts sugary snacks give us, only to leave us depleted and lethargic half an hour later. How about that familiar feeling of still feeling hungry, after finishing off a Chinese takeaway big enough to feed 4 people? This is not a sign of hunger but your body's way of telling you that you did not get all the nutrients from your meal needed to fulfill your appetite, or perhaps that you may be dehydrated. We are all fully aware of the 8 glass a day recommendation for water intake, but not many can say they actually consume that.

Whilst most adopt the opinion of 'everything in moderation' there are certain foods that should not even be eaten in moderation. I believe the majority of people are fully aware of what is good and bad for them. What can be healthier than foods in their natural form, perfectly ripe, full of flavour and put on earth for us by Mother Nature herself?

The human body requires a good balance of healthy foods to be able to function well and achieve a sense of well-being.

Food helps us to:
- Grow
- Reproduce cells to build and repair tissue
- Fight bacteria to avoid disease
- Speed up recovery time from illness

To put it simply, through food we can generally achieve the best of health. Food is the fuel our bodies require to provide the nutrients which create the chemical substances necessary for the functions listed above.

In the past the media has only put the emphasis on obtaining iron from meat and calcium from dairy, forgetting to mention all the plant based foods which also contain iron, protein, calcium and all other vitamins and minerals. Leafy green vegetables such as cabbage, kale, broccoli and spinach contain iron, as well as calcium and protein as do seeds and pulses. Neither is it mentioned that when all nutrients are absorbed through plant based foods, fruit, vegetables, nuts and seeds the risks of disease can be greatly decreased or even extinguished. A Plant based raw diet has been known to prolong the effects of disease contrary to medical belief.

Food in its raw natural state is the perfect food for the human digestive system. Each individual fruit or vegetable has the right amount of enzymes for it to be digested. When the temperature of food is raised above 118 degrees Fahrenheit, enzymes die and vitamins can be depleted. Since digestion depends on enzymes, the body must work harder to produce these lost enzymes in order to process the food.

The human body was not physically designed to eat any kind of animal products, however through the centuries the innate sense of curiosity in society's mind has led to an omnivorous diet. Let us compare our physical structure with that of a carnivorous animal e.g. a dog. A Dog has sharp claws and large canine teeth in order to capture and kill its prey, and then devour it raw; we on the other hand have very delicate hands and small teeth which move in a rotating motion in order to grind nuts and seeds. Constipation, gas, halitosis and heartburn are all caused by meat in the digestive tract. When food is ingested into the colon it is normally broken down and the nutrients absorbed. However processed cooked food, meat and other animal products do not contain enzymes naturally present in raw foods and therefore can not be fully broken down or the nutrients absorbed. When these foods sit in the digestive tract for a long time they begin to putrefy and release more toxins back into the body.

"The end result of today's average diet is a grim but indisputable statistic: The greater the intake of cooked and processed foods and animal products, the greater the occurrence of disease."

Brian Clements - *Living foods for optimum health*

The evidence indicates that a diet without meat and other animal products is typically the way we were designed to live, emphasizing that raw foods are needed either as the complete make-up of one's diet or featured heavily in a healthy cooked diet.

A bit about the Mediterranean Diet

Cyprus is in the North East of the Mediterranean Sea surrounded by Turkey, Israel, Lebanon and Egypt. Its history has seen many civilizations, including Persian, Roman, Arabian, Ottoman and British come and go and conquerors such as Alexander the Great and Cleopatra stake their claim on the small island. It is perfectly understandable that so many would want to keep such a beautiful island to themselves.

According to Greek mythology the very goddess of beauty and love Aphrodite was born at 'Petra tou Romiou' in Paphos Cyprus.
As suggested by some she was born when Uranus (the father of the gods) was castrated by his son Cronus. Cronus threw the severed genitals into the ocean which began to churn and foam. Aphrodite arose from the foam, hence her name which when translated means 'foam born', and the sea carried her to Cyprus.

The warm climate in the Mediterranean makes it ideal for growing vegetables and fruits, which are then eaten in abundance. The vine together with the olive, carob and citrus are probably the oldest and most important trees in Cypriot life. Almost every Greek home has a huge vine covering the courtyard giving ample shade in the summer and plenty of fruit in the autumn. This is where the family sit for meals, socialising and relaxing.

The word Kopiaste is probably as old as the Greek language itself and is often heard when friends meet. In the dictionary you will find the verb kopiasto, meaning: to take the trouble or to strain oneself. But kopiaste, which is the second person plural of this verb has come to mean: 'sit down and share my meal' or 'come sit and let us talk' and as you will soon come to realise socialising and eating are a Greek's favourite pastime.

Greece and Cyprus between them have a vast and plentiful fruit basket. As well as eaten raw, some fruits are dried, others made into wine. What is left over from the wine is often made into Zivania or Tsipouro (the local moon shine) a strong white spirit that will put hair on the chest of anyone brave enough to drink it. It is not my favourite tipple, but on a warm day men are often seen sitting in the shade with a bottle of tsipouro and a couple of shot glasses playing backgammon.

For the Greeks, cuisine is one of the most valued contributions to daily life. A fundamental part of Mediterranean cuisine is the myriad of colourful and flavoursome foods.

At the core of the traditional Greek diet are dark-green leafy vegetables (often picked from the wild), herbs, spices, fresh fruits, vegetables, legumes, nuts, seeds and olive oil which are all consumed in abundance and are high in nutrients and low in animal fats.

All the ingredients in the following table can be put into sweet and savoury dishes, dried or eaten as snacks.

Herbs & Spices	Pulses	Nuts & Seeds	Fruit	Salad & Vegetables
Garlic	Chickpeas	Sesame	Olives &	Tomato
Dill	Lima beans	Pumpkin	their oil	Cucumber
Oregano	Split peas	Sunflower	Lemons	Spinach
Mint	Lentils	Walnuts	Oranges	Red Onions
Coriander	Haricot beans	Almonds	Apricots	Artechokes
Bay Leaves	Black eyed	Pine Nuts	Pomegranites	Fennel
Cinnamon	peas	Pistachios	Prickly Pears	Lettuce
Cumin	Broad beans	Hazelnuts	Figs	Pumpkin
Nutmeg		Poppy	Grapes	Cabbage
Clove			Watermelon	Horta (wild
Flat leaf			Mandarins	greens)
parsley			Peaches	Courgette
Ground black			Nectarines	Bell Peppers
pepper			Carob	Aubergine
			Cherries	Dandelion
			Apples	greens
			Plums	Runner beans
			Pears	Marrow
			Quince	Kolokasi
			Mespilo	Kohlrabi

A typical Greek gathering can sometimes consist of as many as 25 or so dishes (meze), and often starts with a *Village Salad,* bread and *dips,* followed by *yiahni* (marinated in tomato sauce) vegetables like green beans or peas and *rice,* then on to the more heavier foods like a small slice of *moussaka,* or *pastitsio,* and, finally the meat including *koftedes* and *sheftalies* served with *pilafi.* The meal usually ends with fresh chopped fruit and/or vegetables.

The Importance of Greek Cuisine

I was born in London and have lived there all my life. My parents, however, were both born in Cyprus and had typical Greek upbringings. They each brought with them many Greek traditions when they moved to London at different stages of their lives. The most obvious of those traditions is the importance of food and what it represents.

The Greeks love to eat. Ask a Greek about food and their eyes will light up as they animatedly talk of the subject and about how their mothers' cooking is the best. It's not the dish that matters but the taste, the smell, the passion and the pleasure. Life is celebrated with an abundance of food, song and dance. Because the offering and sharing of food is an expression of friendship it is considered impolite to refuse and any occasion is used to host a feast.

A family gathering, which is never less then ten people from my own personal experience, is quite often a huge feast where there is a constant flow of food being served throughout the day. As full as you may be when the next course is served you can always find room for one more slice of cake, some fresh figs, or watermelon and halloumi cheese. You may find it hard to picture this image, you may even think I am exaggerating slightly but I can assure you I never joke when it comes to food. You could compare every Greek get together to Christmas Day where the whole day revolves around eating and drinking. This day may come around once a year for most but imagine if it happened as often as once a week. You can now start to get a feel for what it is like to grow up in a Greek family.

I have always loved food and still do to this day. From a very early age it has been drummed into me that food is important not only for health reasons but also from a social perspective.

The origin of Greek cuisine has been the subject of much debate. Whether Greek cuisine was influenced by neighbouring countries such as Turkey or Israel, or whether those countries have been influenced by Greek cuisine is a mystery to me. However, the fact of the matter is that due to climate the produce is very similar throughout the Mediterranean therefore, the core ingredients are very similar if not the same.

My intention for this book is to incorporate Greek and Cypriot flavours into raw food preparation and adapt many of my favourite cooked meals into raw food interpretations. I have had so much fun experimenting with recipes, ideas and ingredients and am confident that my hard work has created some exquisite dishes. The recipes in this book do not need to be followed precisely as personal taste varies from one person to the next. I think slight variation to recipes makes a dish personal and adds more fun to food preparation. There is a budding chef in all of us. I hope you enjoy this book and have fun following the recipes in it.

'Most of all I hope you relish every mouthful of every dish made.'

My Journey

I would like to think that my whole life has been research for this book. From childhood food has always played a huge part in my life. Being of Greek Cypriot decent I had a good basis for a healthy diet. Fresh fruit and vegetables, pulses, nuts and seeds were all incorporated into my daily food intake and all meals were lovingly prepared with fresh ingredients from scratch, but without too much thought about nutritional content and health. Meats and dairy products although incorporated into our diet never played a huge role and were not a necessity or consumed on a daily basis, purely because that was how my parents were brought up and the traditions were passed down from generation to generation. Without realizing it I was probably already consuming a large amount of raw foods before the concept of the raw food diet was introduced to me. Looking back now I do not remember being sick very often or having to take many, if any days off school due to illness. I now realize a lot of that was down to the healthy way I was eating. As I started to enter adulthood I took more of an interest in food from the diet and weight loss perspective and experimented with many different types of diets. My obsession with food and calories stemmed from a tendency to gain weight very easily, and I guess this is where my interest in nutrition originates.

However in October 2003 I embarked on a long trip to South East Asia, where I met many wonderful people from all around the world and also realized that I was not alone with my obsession with my weight and the fat and calorie content of foods. On my travels I met someone who changed my conscious thoughts towards food for the better. This good friend was the first to suggest a raw food diet to me, leading me to discover the benefits of a vegan diet and why we as a human race are better equipped physically to deal with plant based foods as opposed to animal products and their derivatives. The more I learnt, the more curious I became about the food I was ingesting and the effect it was having on my body internally as well as the differences I was able to see when I looked in the mirror. So for the first time in January 2004 I decided to adopt a vegan diet and was even convinced to try the raw food diet for 3 days. Being in Thailand I was able to feast on huge salads which included water chestnuts, bamboo shoots and sesame seeds plus ate fresh mangos, pineapple, watermelon and drank coconut water straight from the fruit itself.

The list of wonderful, juicy, tasty exotic fruits and vegetables was endless. In that time I spent every day moaning about and wanting noodle soup, Thai green curry and rice, Pad Thai noodles and thinking of all the other things I was going to eat when the 3 days were over. After 3 days, however, I found that I felt no urgency to eat all those things straight away and I was not rushing to the nearest street vendor. From that moment on I was even more inspired and curious, therefore when I got home in March I started to research raw food diets, looking on the internet and reading anything I could lay my eyes on. Eventually I decided to try it for a week as a detox, this ended in me going to a Harmonious Living weekend (two days of raw food, yoga, discussions, learning and socializing), hosted by Ruth Allen, with my mum and her two friends. Here we met Shazzie whose online journal I had been following at the time, Holly Paige who prepared all the wonderful simple yet tasty and filling raw meals and a small group of raw foodists. This was a vital point in my raw journey because after a week of eating 100% raw food I felt great and looked so good again I had no desire to eat anything cooked, cooked food had no appeal whatsoever, even less so than after the 3 days in Thailand. And so my journey into raw food began. Shortly after being back at home in London a friend introduced me to my first experience of the Fresh Festival in Wales where I unexpectedly ended up helping Chad Sarno and his kitchen team for the weekend. I took this opportunity to meet, first hand, raw food advocates such as Doug Graham, Brian Clements, Chad Sarno, Karen Knowler and many more people who, in my eyes, were celebrities and true inspirations to this lifestyle I was now living. I spent the whole weekend helping with the preparation of gourmet raw foods, serving the eager visitors and being inspired by what I heard from guest speakers. I learnt a lot about raw food and how it can be manipulated to look, taste and feel like cooked food but with all the nutrients and benefits of raw food. I was amazed and my taste buds were tantalized. The Fresh Festival was my inspiration for writing this book. Therefore, I hope you enjoy the delights I am presenting you with and please remember that food does not need to be a chore, make it fun and experiment with your own ideas and tastes. Adapt any of these recipes to your personal taste, add or omit ingredients to suit your palate. And remember that once you have mastered the flavours, which come down to mainly the herbs and spices used, the next step is presentation and finally texture. Almost any cooked meal can be adapted with a little patience, experimentation and fun.

In this book I have tried to stick to a basic set of ingredients based on those I know and have grown up enjoying. I have also tried to use ingredients which I know are native to Greece and Cyprus, along with some other ingredients, which are not necessarily locally grown, in order to get the same effects as their cooked alternatives.

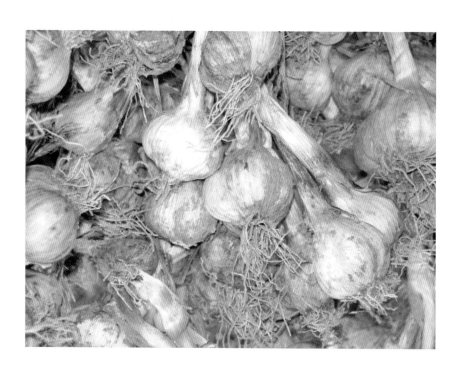

The Recipes

INGREDIENTS

Herbs
Fresh is always best. However, you can buy big bunches of coriander, parsley or mint wash it, make sure it is dry, finely chop and then freeze it. This way you can have fresh herbs as and when they are required. Due to the fact that the herbs have been finely chopped before freezing they do not need to be defrosted before use, just add to the required recipe. You can also dry these herbs in the sun or airing cupboard, again wash and dry them properly before doing so, crumble and store in an airtight container.

Carob powder
This powder comes from pods which grow on trees in hot climates. When ground into a powder it resembles cocoa powder, it is sweet and can be used as a substitute for chocolate. Carob is rich in protein and can be used in drinks, cakes and puddings.

Olives
Olives are often preserved in salt, making them taste very salty. Soak them in water over night to remove the salt, rinsing often where possible and before eating or using in recipes.

Olive Oil
Avoid conventional cooking oils and try to buy stone pressed or cold pressed olive oil. Extra virgin olive oil is considered the best to use; it is extracted from the first pressing of the olives which makes it the least processed.

Salt
Common table salt lacks minerals and trace elements because it has been purified and refined, therefore only use Celtic Sea Salt which has been uniquely harvested preserving its mineral content.

Tahini
Tahini is the butter that has been ground from sesame seeds, in most cases the sesame seeds have been roasted, however raw tahini is available (please see resources page). Tahini is a versatile ingredient, it can be used in soups, dressings, smoothies, desserts, dips etc, its thick creamy texture is very fulfilling and satisfying.

Agave Syrup

Agave syrup is naturally extracted from the inner core of a cactus like plant called Agave which is native to Mexico. Agave syrup is a sweetener and can be compared to honey and maple syrup and used as a replacement for either of these or any other sweetener.

Dried Apricots

When buying dried apricots be sure to buy organic unsulphured apricots, as sulphur can cause allergies. The difference is obvious from their appearance alone; when apricots are unsulphured they become darker with a caramelized, almost fig-like flavour.

Psyllium Husks

Psyllium husks come from the crushed seeds of the Plantago ovata plant, a herb native to parts of Asia, Mediterranean regions of Europe and North Africa. Psyllium is similar to oats and wheat and is rich in soluble fiber. Psyllium can be found in any health food store. In raw food cuisine it is often used as a thickening agent.

Tamari

Tamari is similar to Soy sauce, it is also derived from soya beans, but from the process used to make miso. Therefore, it is fermented and exposed to certain microbiological cultures and aged in salt producing a tasty, dark red paste. Tamari is a live food if unpastuerised. The word Tamari, means 'that which accumulates' this is because the protein-rich liquid accumulates during the miso ripening process.

Flax Seed Oil

Flaxseeds are also called linseeds and are best known for the therapeutic oil that is derived by pressing them. The nutty Flax seed oil is considered to be nature's richest source of essential fatty acids (EFA's).

Apple Cider Vinegar

I would suggest using Bragg's Organic Apple Cider Vinegar because it is unfiltered, unheated and unpasteurized, making it a raw product. Made from apples this zesty vinegar has been highly regarded throughout history for its amazing health qualities. Rich in enzymes and potassium it has been said that Hippocrates used it as an antibiotic.

Sprouting

Freshly sprouted seeds and beans are considered a living food because the dormant seed or bean springs to life. By soaking, draining and leaving seeds to germinate and sprout the nutritional value and digestibility is greatly increased. Sprouts are rich in essential nutrients, vitamins, minerals, Amino Acids, proteins and phytochemicals.

English/American translations

Courgette = Zucchini
Aubergine = Eggplant
Coriander = Cilantro
Spring onions = Green Onions
Chick peas = Garbanzos
Pepper = Bell pepper
Rocket = Arugula

EQUIPMENT

When it comes to buying equipment shop around, ask friends opinions or even try to borrow someone elses juicer for example, this way you can get a real feel for the limitations of the equipment you want to buy. Everybody has an opinion and a reason for liking or disliking something and due to the fact that some of the equipment mentioned below is expensive, you want to be sure you get your moneys worth. I have made some suggestions below but new items appear on the market all the time, so don't just take my word for it.

Dehydrator
Dehydrators can be very expensive and time consuming when it comes to preparing raw food. For these reasons purchasing one was not a priority when I was transitioning into a raw food diet. Because of this I tried to create recipes that did not require a dehydrator however, due to the fact that I am imitating cooked food in some cases it was almost impossible to avoid therefore a few recipes do call for a dehydrator.
A dehydrator is a piece of equipment which blows warm (not hot) air over the food so that some of the moisture is removed and the food dried. Due to the fact that the temperature is kept low the enzymes and nutrients are not lost as they would normally be in an oven. If, however, you have not yet got around to buying a dehydrator you can achieve the same results using your oven on its lowest temperature and leaving the door open slightly, alternatively you can use the sun or the airing cupboard to dehydrate food.

There are currently a few dehydrators on the market, however, I would recommend the Excalibur dehydrator, it is front loading like an oven for ease of use and has a heat gauge which allows you to control the temperature.

Juicers
Juicing fresh fruit and vegetables can have endless health benefits, a juicer is one of the most important pieces of equipment to have in one's kitchen. There are many juicers on the market at the moment ranging from between £40 and £400+ making buying a juicer a very hard decision to make. The Champion juicer is one of the most popular amongst raw foodists, it is also one of the most expensive. The reason for its popularity is its versatility, it can be used for juicing wheatgrass and by using the homogenizer it can make nut cheeses and turn frozen bananas into

ice-cream. In my experience, however, I have found that the Samson can do exactly the same job and is slightly cheaper and much easier to clean.

Citrus juicers are also a great tool to have in your kitchen for a quick glass of freshness or when preparing food where lemon juice is a big feature (as is the case in Mediterranean cuisine). Citrus juicers are relatively cheap and can be found in department stores or kitchen accessory retailers.

Mandoline & Spiral slicer

The mandoline is a handy gadget and has been my secret weapon when it comes to making raw food look more like cooked dishes. It is a simple to use manual gadget that perfectly slices fruit and vegetables thick and thin. By using other blades you can also julienne, shred or grate vegetables. The spiral slicer is a similar gadget which can create pasta-like noodles out of courgettes, carrots and most hard vegetables. Depending on your preference I strongly suggest buying one or the other of these gadgets.

Blender

Any blender can be used to make smoothies, soups, sauces and salad dressings and a lot of standard blenders come with a coffee mill which I think is very useful for grinding spices or milling seeds and nuts into flour. The Vitamix, which is also very popular with raw foodists however gets the smoothest results. The Vitamix is a high powered blender that can pulverize anything hard or soft into a very smooth texture but again it is an expensive piece of equipment.

Food Processor

If you have a Vitamix you would probably have little need for a food processor, however, if you only have a standard blender you may find a food processor more convenient when pulverizing hard things such as nuts, or hard vegetables such as carrots. Some food processors also come with extra attachments which can be used for grating or slicing. When I first started eating a raw food diet I used my food processor for everything because I did not have a blender. I now use it for the more heavy duty processing, like nuts or hard vegetables like parsnips, and I use my blender for smoothies.

See the resources page for listings of suppliers etc.

"An apple a day keeps the doctor away."

Your Mother

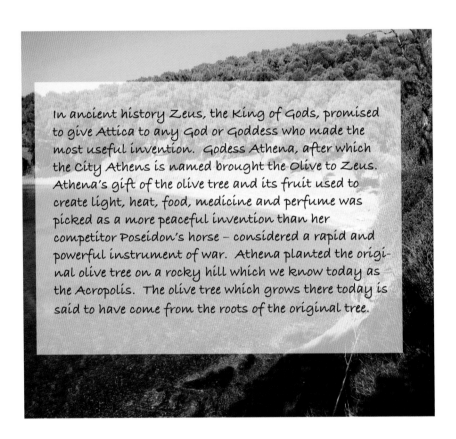

In ancient history Zeus, the King of Gods, promised to give Attica to any God or Goddess who made the most useful invention. Godess Athena, after which the City Athens is named brought the Olive to Zeus. Athena's gift of the olive tree and its fruit used to create light, heat, food, medicine and perfume was picked as a more peaceful invention than her competitor Poseidon's horse – considered a rapid and powerful instrument of war. Athena planted the original olive tree on a rocky hill which we know today as the Acropolis. The olive tree which grows there today is said to have come from the roots of the original tree.

APPETIZERS

Meze Vegetables
Marinated Olives
Elies Tsakistes
'Sautéed' Mushrooms
Marinated Beetroot

Meze Vegetables

Artichokes - Anginares

The artichoke is eaten raw. In order to do so, you only eat the bottom and the small white part at the end of each leaf. Wash it well, and then pull off all the leaves. The bottom is cleaned of the choke (the hairy part in the middle) and the stringy parts on the outside, then rubbed with plenty of lemon to keep it white, cut into quarters or eight parts and serve as a meze with lemon and salt.

Cabbage - Krambi

The local cabbage in both Greece and Cyprus is larger, crisper and smaller then its European cousin. It is only eaten raw, cut finely and dressed with lemon juice, salt and olive oil.

Kohlrabi - Kouloumbres

They are eaten only raw, peeled and cut into segments and dressed in lemon juice and salt

Many other vegetables can be dressed in lemon juice, salt and sometimes olive oil depending on the vegetable i.e. carrots, cucumber tomatoes etc.

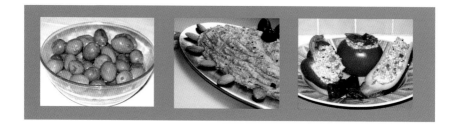

Marinated Olives

- 2 cups kalamata olives soaked overnight and rinsed thoroughly
* *Black sun dried olives can also be used although kalamata olives work best.*
- 2 tbsp lemon zest
- 2 cloves of garlic crushed
- 2 tbsp olive oil
- 1 tbsp fresh minced rosemary
- 2 tbsp lemon juice

1 In a bowl mix the lemon juice and zest with the crushed garlic, olive oil and rosemary. Mix thoroughly until the olive oil has been mixed well with the other ingredients.

2 Place the olives in a container and pour the marinade over them stirring to ensure all the olives are covered

3 Cover the olives and place in a cool dry place, not the fridge, for between a couple of hours or a few days depending on how strong you want them to taste.

Elies Tsakistes

Crushed Olives

*This recipe takes approximately 30 days to complete

'Olives & Brine (Part 1)'
- 4 glasses of water
- 4 tbsp Celtic sea salt
* *Stir well so that the salt dissolves.*
- 400g raw green olives
(Part 2)
- 3 tbsp olive oil
- 2 cloves garlic crushed
- 1tsp Celtic sea salt
- Lemon Juice
- 2 tbsp pounded coriander seeds
- 3 cloves lightly crushed garlic
- A slice or 2 of lemon finely chopped

1 Crush the olives – using a hammer put the olives in a plastic bag and ensure all the olives are bashed at least once. Thoroughly rinse and soak in water for about 15 hours.

2 Wash the olives very well, changing their water 2-3 times and drain. Put them in a jar, add the lemon juice (for 400g of olives add 1 tbsp lemon juice) and enough brine to cover them.

3 Finally add the olive oil, its height in the jar must be about 1cm and it must be 3-4 cm below the lid of the jar. The olives should be ready in about 20-30 days or when the bitterness has gone

4 After the olives have been allowed to soak for a substantial amount of time and the bitterness has more or less gone, drain, rinse them thoroughly and set aside.

5 In another bowl mix together the coriander seeds, salt, garlic and 2 tbsp lemon juice, poor over the olives mix together well until all the olives are covered. Throw the lemon pieces in last and lightly toss. Place the olives in an airtight container and store in the fridge for a couple of days. The olives are then ready to be served.

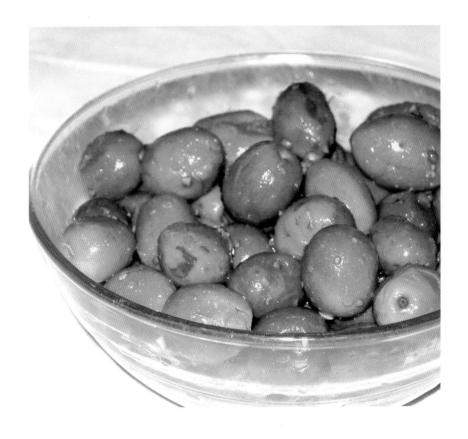

'Sautéed' Mushrooms

Serve as a side dish, or add to other recipes

- 250g button mushrooms finely chopped
- 1 red onion finely chopped
- 4 tbsp olive oil
- 8 tbsp parsley finely chopped
- 1 lemon juiced
- Add salt if desired

Add all the ingredients to a flat bottomed bowl and mix together well, let marinade over night until the mushrooms become soft.

Marinated Beetroot

Serve as a side dish, or add to other recipes

- 4 fresh beetroot bulbs finely chopped into cubes
- half a glass of fresh lemon juice (approximately 1 lemon)
- 4 tbsp olive oil
- $1/2$ tsp sea salt
- 2 tbsp fresh thyme or 1 tbsp dry thyme

Add all the ingredients to a flat bottomed bowl and mix together well, let marinade for a few hours or over night, or until the beetroot takes on the flavour of the herbs.

"Let food be thy medicine, and let thy medicine be food."

Hippocrates

DIPS

Olive Spread
Tashi
Houmus
Tzatziki

Olive Spread

- 1 2/3 cups kalamata olives pitted and soaked overnight
- 2 1/4 cups almonds soaked overnight
- 3 tbsp olive oil
- 1/2 - 3/4 cup lemon juice
- 2 cloves garlic crushed
- 2 tbsp capers

1 Rinse the almonds and grind in a food processor until they are finely chopped. Set aside in a bowl.

2 Put the olives in the food processor with the capers and blend until the olives have also been finely processed.

3 Add the remaining ingredients to the food processor including the almonds and process until all the ingredients are thoroughly mixed together; you may have to do this in 2 batches in order for the ingredients to be mixed together thoroughly.

4 You may add more lemon juice, capers, or garlic depending on your personal taste.

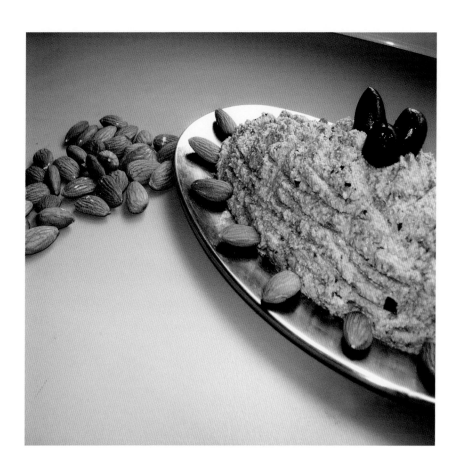

Tashi

Sesame dip

- 1 cup raw tahini
- 1 - 1$^{1/2}$ level tsp Celtic sea salt
- 10-11 tbsp fresh lemon juice
- 1-2 cloves crushed garlic
- $^{3/4}$ cup water

In a food processor place the tahini, salt and garlic, while this is mixing add the lemon juice, once this is all gone slowly add the water a little at a time, being very careful not to put too much water (once there is too much water it is impossible to rectify). Once the tahini becomes light and grayish in colour, and smooth and thick in texture it is ready. Remove from the food processor, place in a dish cover and chill until ready to be served.

Houmus

Chick pea dip

- 1 cup sprouted chick peas
- 1 - 2 lemons juiced depending on how juicy they are
  and personal taste.
- 2 tbsp raw tahini
- 3 tbsp olive oil
- 1 clove crushed garlic
- Celtic sea salt to taste

Place all the ingredients into a food processor and process until smooth.
Depending on your taste you can add more or less lemon juice.

Tzatziki

'Yogurt' & Cucumber dip

- 2 avocadoes
- 3 tbsp crushed dry mint
- half an onion shredded in a mandoline or finely diced
- 2 garlic cloves crushed
- 1 cucumber shredded in a mandoline or finely diced
- 6 tbsp lemon juice or more if desired
- 1 tsp Celtic sea salt
- 1/2 tsp fresh ground pepper

1 Shred the cucumber and lay on some kitchen towel to draw out the excess water whilst preparing the other ingredients.

2 Cut the avocadoes in half remove the seed, scoop out the flesh and place in the food processor along with the salt, pepper, lemon juice and garlic. Blend together until the avocado is smooth.

3 Place the avocado mix in a bowl with the cucumber, onion and mint and mix.

" Health is the greatest gift,
contentment the greatest wealth, faithful-
ness the best relationship."

Buddha

Raw salads are a matter of creativity and imagination. A great salad can be made from the various seasonal vegetables to be found at the green grocers.

Grate some white or red cabbage, chop a little lettuce, some carrots, spring onions, dill or parsley, slice a leek, add a little uncooked spinach, rocket, a pepper or two of any colour and or whatever else comes to mind. Mix together; add salt, black pepper, perhaps some tomatoes, cucumber and pure virgin olive oil.

A meal in minutes in my opinion.

SALADS

Horiatiki
Artabio Original
Red Cabbage
'Rice'
Pilafi
Melitzanosalata

Dressings
Greek
Tahini
Almond

Horiatiki

Village Salad

- 2 beef tomatoes or 3 normal tomatoes
- Half a large cucumber
- 1 green pepper
- 1 red onion
- 5 black olives
- 1 tbsp dried oregano

'Dressing'
- 2 tbsp olive oil
- Celtic sea salt to taste
- Freshly ground pepper to taste
- Juice of half a lemon

Chop and place all the ingredients in a bowl and lightly toss in the dressing and sprinkle with oregano.

Artabio Original

- 1 head of romaine lettuce
- 1 red onion
- 2 oranges peeled
- A handful of hulled walnuts

'Dressing'
- 1 tbsp olive oil
- Celtic sea salt
- Pepper
- Juice of 1 lemon

Chop and place all the ingredients apart from the walnuts in a bowl, add the dressing and toss. Roughly crush and sprinkle the walnuts over the top of the salad and serve.

"This recipe was put together during my stay at a farm in Arta Greece during the spring of 2005. Not much was in season at the time so we had to improvise with the ingredients we had, collectively we all came up with this salad, surprisingly it tasted very good."

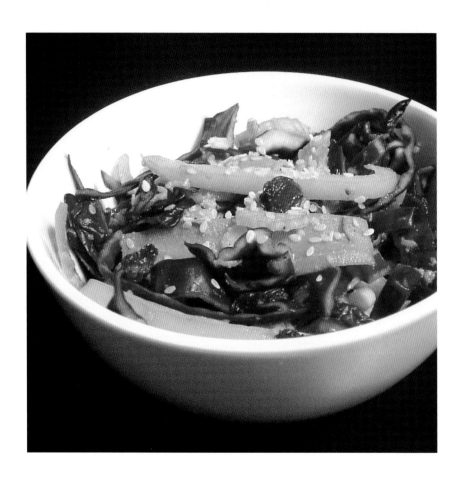

Red Cabbage Salad

- 1 red cabbage shredded
- 2 large carrots grated
- 5 spring onions finely chopped
- 1 grated apple
- 1 yellow pepper finely sliced
- half a cup of sultanas soaked for 6 hours

'Dressing'
- 1 $^{1/2}$ tbsp tahini
- 2 tbsp apple cider vinegar
- 1 lemon juiced
- 1 tsp Celtic sea salt
- $1/2$ tsp freshly ground pepper
- 1 tbsp sesame seeds

Place all the ingredients in a bowl. Mix together the dressing and pour over the salad. Toss and serve.

'Rice'

- 6 parsnips peeled and roughly chopped
- 2 carrots finely chopped
- 3/4 cup red cabbage finely shredded
- 6 sticks of celery finely chopped
- 1 1/2 cups pine nuts
- 1 cup dried unsulphured apricots (soaked for 2 hours)
- 4 tbsp sesame seeds
- 8 tbsp flax seed oil
- 1/2 cup lemon juice
- 2 tsp Celtic sea salt
- 4 tbsp fresh parsley finely chopped
- 1 tsp freshly ground pepper

1 Peel and roughly chop the parsnips, place in the food processor and pulse until it is chopped and resembles rice a little in consistency

2 Remove the parsnip from the food processor and place in a large bowl, put the pine nuts in the processor and pulse until they are roughly chopped and add to the bowl

3 Add the remaining ingredients to the bowl mix together and serve.

Pilafi

Cous Cous Salad

- 1 cauliflower roughly chopped
- 3 spring onions sliced
- 1 red pepper finely cut
- 1 cup raisins soaked for 2 hours
- 1 tsp turmeric
- 1 tsp cumin
- 2 tbsp flaxseed oil
- Sautéed mushrooms (page 26)

1 Put the cauliflower in the food processor and pulse until its consistency becomes like cous cous. Place in a bowl.

2 Drain and rinse the raisins and place in the bowl with the remaining ingredients, including the 'Sautéed' mushrooms. Toss well and serve.

Melitzanosalata

Aubergine Salad

- 3 large aubergines
- 1/2 cup of olive oil
- 3 cloves of garlic crushed
- 3/4 cup lemon juice
- 3 tbsp chopped parsley
- 1 tsp salt
- 1/2 tsp fresh ground pepper

1 Shred the aubergines using the mandoline and soak in salt water over night.

2 After soaking the aubergine strain off the water and cut into small piece.

3 In a bowl mix the lemon juice, parsley, salt, pepper, and olive oil and add the aubergine. Mix together thoroughly and serve with a sprig of parsley

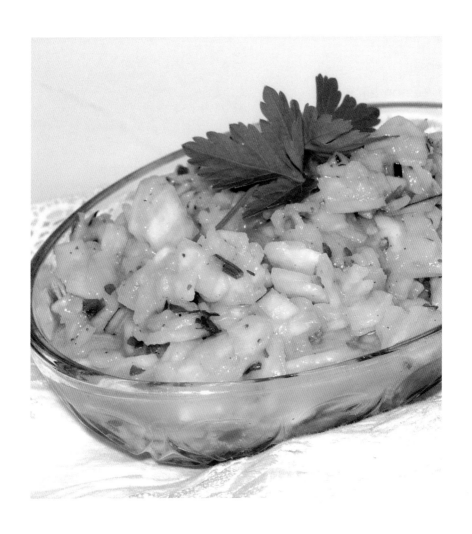

Salad Dressings

Basic Greek Salad Dressing

- Olive Oil
- Salt
- Lemon Juice

These ingredients can be added to any salad, in the quantities best preferred. Some people prefer their salads with plenty of olive oil, others like more of a lemony taste.

Tahini Dressing

- 2 tablespoons tahini
- 1/4 cup fresh orange juice (roughly half an orange)
- 1/2 tsp sea salt
- 1/2 tsp fresh ground pepper
- 1/4 teaspoon cinnamon

Place all the ingredients into the blender and blend together. This dressing is best served with simple salad vegetables, like lettuce, cucumber, carrots

Almond Dressing

- $1/2$ cup raw almonds soaked overnight
- $1/2$ lemon juiced
- 1 cup water
- 1 tbsp raw agave syrup
- $1/2$ tsp pepper
- 1 tbsp fresh basil chopped
- 1 clove garlic crushed

Firstly grind the almonds with a little water in the food processor. Once the almonds have been ground to a pulp add all the other ingredients including the rest of the water. You can add a little water at a time until you get a consistency you like.

This dressing tastes sensational without salt, however you may want to add some once you have added it to a salad.

Shiny yellow lemons add a bright splash to every market and table spread. They can be served with practically every meze or vegetable dish. The acidity reduces the heaviness of the olive oil.

To maximize the amount of juice squeezed out of a lemon, it should be brought to room temperature or rolled under the palm of your hand on a flat surface before slicing.

FINGER FOODS

Dolmadakia
Koftedes
Kolokotes
Sheftalies
Stuffed Tomatoes

Dolmadakia

Stuffed Vine Leaves

'Vine leaves'
- 30 fresh vine leaves
- 2 lemons juiced
- 5 tbsp olive oil
- 2 tsp Celtic sea salt

'Filling'
- 3 cups parsnip (approximately 4 parsnips)
- 3/4 cup pine nuts
- 4 medium tomatoes
- 1 tbsp olive oil
- 6 tbsp lemon juice
- 1 tsp Celtic sea salt
- 1/2 tsp freshly ground pepper
- 1/2 medium red onion
- 2 tbsp fresh mint or 1 tbsp dry mint

1 Mix all the ingredients for the marinade. Dip each individual vine leaf into the marinade ensuring both sides are covered, stack and lay them aside pouring over the left over marinade and let marinade for about 5-6 hours.

2 Peel and chop the parsnips and process until it becomes similar to rice in consistency. Remove the parsnip and place in a bowl.

3 Put the pine nuts in the food processor and process until they also become like rice in consistency and add to the bowl with the parsnips.

4 Process 2 of the 4 tomatoes so they are liquified and add to the bowl.

5 Finely chop the other 2 tomatoes and the onion, chop or crumble the mint (depending if fresh or dry) and add to the bowl along with the olive oil, salt and pepper. Mix all the ingredients together thoroughly.

6 Take a vine leaf and place onto a flat surface so the stork side is facing up and is closest to you.

7 Place a tablespoon of mixture in the middle of the leaf, from the bottom of the leave (closest to you) fold it over the mixture once followed by each side and roll up the remaining leaf pressing firmly to ensure the filling stays in place.

Makes approximately 30 stuffed vine leaves

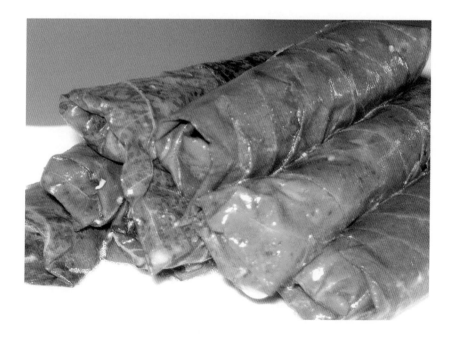

Koftedes

'Meat' balls

- 4 cups walnuts (soaked for 2 hours)
- 1-1$^{1/2}$ cup parsley finely chopped
- $^{1/2}$ cup mint chopped
- 2 cups onion finely chopped (app 2 large)
- 3 cups sweet potato grated (app 3)
- 1 large courgette half shredded in a mandoline and then finely chopped
- 6 sun dried tomatoes (soaked for 2 hours)
- 6 tbsp fresh lemon juice
- 2 tbsp olive oil
- 1 tsp Celtic sea salt

1 In a food processor blend together the walnuts, half the sweet potato, half the onion and the un-shredded courgette, plus the lemon juice, olive oil, salt and sun dried tomatoes until smooth.

2 Place the blended mixture in a bowl and add the remaining ingredients, mix well.

3 Form mixture into small balls about 1.5 inches in diameter and dehydrate for approximately 8 hours.

Makes approximately 50 balls

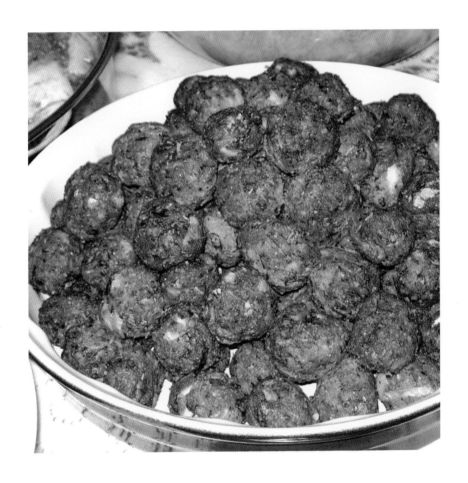

Kolokotes

Pumpkin Pies

- 8 courgettes

- 1 small butternut squash

- 1 small cauliflower

- 2 tbsp olive oil

- 1 tsp Celtic sea salt

- 1 $1/2$ tsp fresh ground pepper

- 1 $1/2$ tsp cinnamon

- 1 cup raisins (soaked for 2 hours)

- 3 tbsp flax seed oil

1 Thinly slice the courgettes using a mandoline, sprinkle with salt and let sweat for an hour while preparing the rest of the ingredients.

2 Peel and grate the squash and place in a bowl

3 Chop the cauliflower into chunks and process until its consistency becomes similar to cous cous. Add to the bowl with the squash.

4 In the bowl with the cauliflower and squash add the oil, raisins, salt, pepper and cinnamon and mix together.

5 Take 2 strips of courgette and lay one on top of the other in a cross shape. Place a large teaspoon of mixture in the centre press down into a ball fold the courgette strips over to form small cubed like parcels.

6 Place parcels in the dehydrator for about 4 hours until the courgette has shrunk a little. Do not leave them in there too long or they will begin to taste too salty.

Makes approximately 45 parcels

Sheftalies
'Sausages'

- 1 red pepper finely chopped
- 1 green pepper finely chopped
- 4 cups walnuts (soaked for 2 hours)
- 1 cup parsley finely chopped
- 2 cups onion finely chopped
- 6 sun dried tomatoes (soaked for 2 hours)
- 3 cups mushrooms finely chopped
- 1 cups fresh tomatoes finely chopped
- 6 tbsp fresh lemon juice
- 2 tbsp olive oil
- 2 tsp Celtic sea salt
- 1 1/2 tsp fresh ground pepper
- 1/2 tsp freshly ground cinnamon

1 Firstly dress the mushrooms in 2 tbsp olive oil, 6 tbsp lemon juice, 1 tbsp finely chopped parsley and half a tsp salt, mix thoroughly so all the mushrooms are covered in the marinade and let stand for 2 hours.

2 In another bowl put the onions, the remaining parsley, tomatoes and peppers.

3 Once the walnuts have been soaking for 2 hours drain, rinse process and add to the bowl with the other ingredients including the mushrooms, olive oil, remaining salt, pepper and cinnamon.

4 Once thoroughly mixed together, take a small amount of the mixture and mould into a small sausage shape about 2 inches in length and 1 inch in width, and dehydrate for approximately 8 hours or until the the coating is relatively solid and the 'sausages' have changed colour.

Makes approximately 50 'sausages'

Stuffed Tomatoes

- 1 cup raw pumpkin seeds soaked for 6 hours

- 1 cup raw sunflower seeds soaked for 6 hours

- 1/2 medium red onion

- 2 tbsp tamari

- 1/2 cup coarsely chopped fresh basil

- 1/4 teaspoon freshly ground black pepper

- 1/2 tsp salt

- 1 lemon juiced

- Approximately 40 small tomatoes on the vine

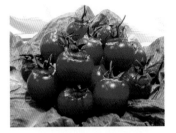

1 Drain and thoroughly rinse the seeds draining thoroughly one last time. Put the seeds and the rest of the ingredients (apart from the tomatoes) into the food processor and process until smooth.

2 Carefully cut the tomatoes from the vines using scissors so that the stalk remains on the tomato tops. Wipe them clean with a damp cloth and dry with kitchen towel.

3 Carefully slice the tops of the tomatoes so that the stalks do not fall off. Scoop out the seeds from inside the tomato with a small spoon, being careful not to break the tomato shell.

4 Gently stuff the tomatoes with the seed mix, place the tops back on and serve.

Olives have been cultivated in Greece since ancient times. For centuries olive oil has been regarded as a gift from the Gods by the ancient Greeks. Olive trees were high in value, the value of one's land was measured by the amount of olive trees that grew on it. The first time the olives are pressed the golden green oil known as extra virgin olive oil is extracted and it is used in the majority of most traditional Greek dishes. As well as being used for their richly flavored oil, olives are commonly eaten whole, as a side dish and also put into bread.

The nutritional value of olive oil is high due to the numerous health benefits attributed to it. It is high in monounsaturated fat and studies have shown that it raises levels of HDL (high-density lipoprotein) i.e. 'good' cholesterol while lowering artery-clogging LDL (low-density lipoprotein) i.e. 'bad' cholesterol. People who eat a diet high in monounsaturated fat, such as the traditional Greek diet, are known to have a lower risk of heart disease than those who eat lots of saturated fats, e.g. butter, margarine and other animal fats.

MAINS

Moussaka
Rouvithi
Spanakopita
Pastitio
Yiahni
Barayemista

Moussaka

Layered Vegetables with a creamy sauce

'Layered Vegetables'
- 1 aubergine peeled and finely sliced using a mandoline
- 1 courgette finely sliced using a mandoline
- 10 large button mushrooms
- 6 carrots grated
- 1 tsp Celtic sea salt

'Mincemeat'
- 2 small or 1 medium red onion
- 2 tomatoes
- 4 tbsp olive oil
- 1 tsp Celtic sea salt
- 1 tbsp parsley finely chopped
- 1 lemon juiced
- 1 garlic clove crushed

'Crema'
- 1 cup pine nuts
- 1/2 cup hulled sesame seeds soaked
- 1/2 cup almonds soaked and peeled
- 1/2 tsp salt
- 6 tbsp orange juice
- 1/2 cup water
- 1/2-1 tsp cinnamon
- 1/2-1 tsp nutmeg
- 2 tsp agave syrup

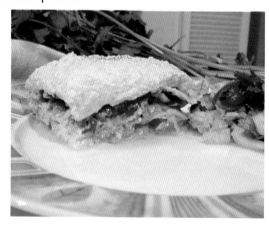

1 Finely slice the aubergine and courgette using a mandoline. Lay some kitchen towel on a plate, or tray and layer the aubergine and courgette sprinkling each layer with a little sea salt. Set aside for a few hours to let them sweat in order to take away the bitter taste.

2 Slice the mushrooms thinly using a knife, the stalks and pieces which are too fiddly to slice set aside. Marinate the slices in the juice of 1/2 lemon 2 tbsp olive oil and 1/4 tsp sea salt, set aside and let marinade for a few hours.

3 Finely chop the remainder of the mushrooms, onion and tomato and marinate in 2 tbsp olive oil, 1/4 tsp sea salt, the juice of half a lemon, 1 tbsp parsley and 1 clove of garlic crushed. Once all the vegetables have been marinating for at least 2 hours, grate the carrots, place in a bowl and pour the marinade from the sliced mushrooms over the carrot and mix together well.

4 In a 6.5" x 8.5" flat bottom glass dish layer half the courgette slices, followed by the sliced mushrooms, grated carrot, half of the aubergine slices, "mincemeat" and finish off with the other half of the courgette slices, and the other half of the aubergine slices. Place in the fridge.

5 Blend the pine nuts, sesame seeds and almonds until smooth, add the remaining ingredients from the 'crema' list, and smooth the mixture on top of the vegetables. Leave the whole dish to chill in the fridge for 30-60 minutes before serving.

6 Before serving sprinkle with a dusting of cinnamon or garnish with a sprig of parsley and serve with a nice "Greek Salad".

Rouvithi

Chick peas & Spinach

- 150g spinach leaves.
- 1 cup chick peas sprouted
- 4 tbsp olive oil
- 1/4 cup lemon juice
- 1 medium onion finely diced
- 1 tsp Celtic sea salt

Place all the ingredients in a bowl and massage together. Set aside (outside of the fridge) for an hour or so until the spinach has softened.

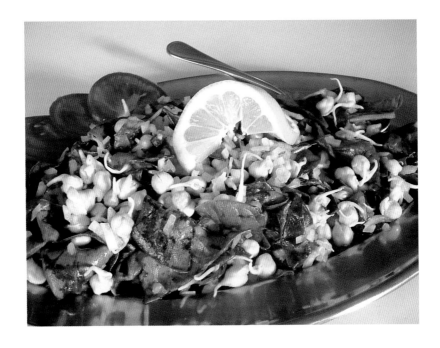

Spanakopita

Spinach pie

'Filling'
- 2 cups spinach
- 2 cups shredded spinach
- 5 spring onions cut finely
- $^{1/2}$ cup chopped parsley
- 2 tbsp dry mint
- 1 cup pine nuts
- 1 tbsp olive oil
- 1 tsp Celtic sea salt

'Pastry'
- 2 courgettes
- 1 tsp Celtic sea salt

1 Thinly slice the courgettes using a mandoline, sprinkle with salt and let sweat (this removes the bitter taste) for an hour while preparing the rest of the ingredients.

2 Put the uncut spinach in the food processor with the pine nuts, olive oil and salt and process until smooth.

3 Rinse the sliced courgette and lay on some kitchen towel to absorb the excess water.

4 Place 2 layers of courgette flat in the bottom of a 6.5" x 8.5" glass dish spread the spinach mixture on top and cover with another 2 layers of courgette. Place the whole dish in the dehydrator at 118°F for 4 hours, until the courgette has shrunk.

Pastitsio

'Macaroni' with a creamy sauce

'Macaroni'
- 3 courgettes finely shredded using a mandoline
- 1 tsp Celtic sea salt
- 4 tbsp olive oil
- 1 cup black olives soaked for 8 hours (changing the water frequently) thoroughly rinsed and pitted

'Mincemeat'
- 2 small or 1 medium red onion finely chopped
- 250g button mushrooms finely chopped
- 2 tomatoes finely chopped
- 4 tbsp olive oil
- 2 tbsp fresh parsley finely chopped
- 1 tbsp fresh mint finely chopped
- 1/4 cup lemon juice
- 1 clove garlic crushed
- 1 tsp Celtic sea salt
- 1/4 tsp freshly ground pepper

'Crema'
- 1 cup pine nuts
- 1/2 cup hulled sesame seeds soaked
- 1/2 cup almonds soaked and peeled
- 1/2 tsp salt
- 6 tbsp orange juice
- 1/2 cup water
- 1/2-1 tsp cinnamon
- 1/2-1 tsp nutmeg
- 2 tsp agave syrup

1 Lay the shredded courgette on some kitchen towel and liberally sprinkle with Celtic sea salt. Set aside for a few hours to release the excess water and soften the courgette.

2 Meanwhile in a bowl put all the ingredients from the 'mince-meat' list and mix together. Set aside and let marinade for a few hours.

3 Once all the other vegetables have been marinating for a few hours, finely chop the olives. Rinse the courgette and lay on kitchen towel for 5 minutes to absorb the excess water. Place in a bowl with the olive oil and a 1/4 tsp salt and mix together.

4 In a round flat bottom dish approximately 8" in diameter place half the courgette and flatten down. On top of the courgette put the 'mincemeat' mix followed by the chopped olives. Finally add the other half of the courgette and flatten down in the dish. Place the whole dish in the fridge.

5 Blend the pine nuts, sesame seeds and almonds until smooth, add the remaining ingredients from the 'crema' list, and smooth the mixture on top of the courgette. Leave the whole dish to chill in the fridge for 30-60 minutes before serving.
Before serving sprinkle with a dusting of cinnamon or garnish with a sprig of parsley and serve with a "Greek Salad".

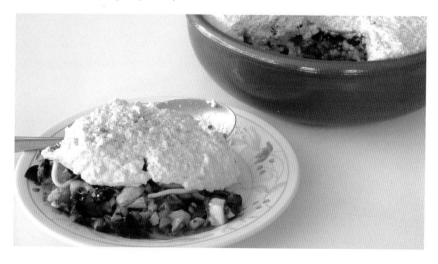

Yiahni

Vegetables with Tomato

500g of any of the following
- Okra - Bamia
- French beans – Fasolaki
- Shelled peas – Bizeli

* Ensure that when you buy the vegetables they are soft and fresh.

- 1/4 tsp Celtic sea salt
- 1/4 tsp pepper
- 2 large tomatoes on the vine
- 1 large red onion
- 4 tbsp olive oil
- 1/4 cup lemon juice
- 2 cloves of garlic

French Beans

Top and tail and cut in half if they are long, or to your desired length.

Okra

Top and tail but only take off a small amount from both ends. This vegetable has a tendency to become slimey if cut in half, therefore keep whole.

Place all the ingredients in a bowl and mix well let stand at room temperature for an hour or so until the vegetables soften a little.

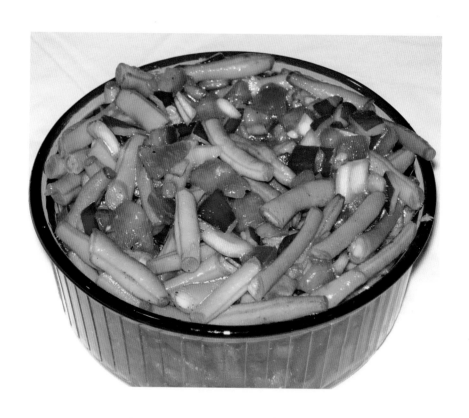

Barayemista

Stuffed Vegetables

'Vegetables for stuffing'
- 1 red pepper
- 1 green pepper
- 1 courgette
- 2 beef tomatoes

'Filling'
- 3 cups parsnip (approximately 4 parsnips)
- 3/4 cup pine nuts
- 4 medium tomatoes
- 1 tbsp olive oil
- 6 tbsp lemon juice
- 1 tsp Celtic sea salt
- 1/2 tsp freshly ground pepper
- 1/2 medium red onion
- 2 tbsp fresh mint or 1 tbsp dry mint

1 Peel and chop the parsnips and process until it becomes similar to rice in consistency. Remove the parsnip and place in a bowl.

2 Put the pine nuts in the food processor and process until they also become like rice in consistency and add to the bowl with the parsnips.

3 Process and liquify 2 of the 4 tomatoes and add to the bowl.

4 Finely chop the other 2 tomatoes and the onion, chop or crumble the mint (depending if fresh or dry) and add to the bowl along with the olive oil, salt and pepper. Mix all the ingredients together thoroughly.

5 Cut the tops off the tomatoes to be stuffed and spoon out the middle adding to the bowl containing the filling.

6 Slice the courgette in half length ways and scoop out the middle, finely chop the part that has been removed and add to the filling.

7 Cut the peppers in half lengthways and dispose of the seeds, or chop the tops off and scoop out the seeds.

8 Stuff the vegetables with the "rice" mixture and serve

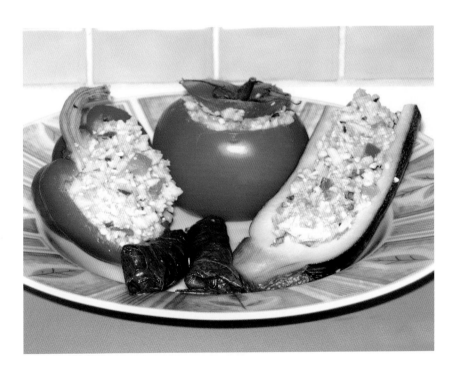

Carob pod, also called St. John's Bread, has been consumed since ancient times and is refereed to in the Bible. It is said that St. John sustained himself for long periods of time on the nutrition of the carob fruit.

SWEETS

Melomacarouna
Peach & Apricot Pie
Orange & Fig 'Crema'
Halva
Cinnamon Biscuits
Plum Pudding

Melomacarouna

'Honey' Cakes

*Makes approximately 20 cakes
- 1 cup agave syrup
- 1 cup fresh Orange Juice
- 4 cups ground almonds soaked overnight
- 1/2 cup of golden flax seeds ground
- 2 tbsp orange rind
- 2 tsp cinnamon
- 4 medjool dates
- 1 tsp Celtic sea salt
- Crushed walnuts for decorating

1 Put the dates through the juicer and then place in the blender with the agave syrup, orange juice and zest. Blend together until all the ingredients are well mixed.

2 Drain and rinse the almonds and feed through the juicer with the blank blade. Place in the food processor with the ground flaxseed, cinnamon and salt and very briefly pulsate

3 Put the agave, dates, orange rind and the orange juice into the blender and mix until the dates have disintegrated and the mixture has all mixed well.

4 Pour some of the liquid from the blender into the food processor and process while adding more liquid a little at a time until it all starts to bind and the mixture is evenly mixed together.

5 Take small pieces of the mixture and with your hands form into oval biscuit shapes and place onto a dehydrator tray.

6 Crush or lightly grind the walnuts and sprinkle on top of the biscuits and place in the dehydrator on 118°F for about 3 hours and then at 100°F for 2 hours.

* These cakes should be slightly crispy on the outside but soft and moist on the inside.

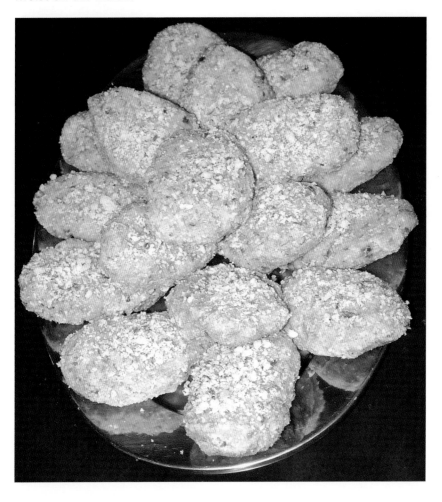

Peach & Apricot Pie

'Base'
- 2 cups almonds soaked
- 1 cup pecans soaked
- 1 cup pitted dates
- 1 orange juiced
- 3 inch piece of vanilla pod

'Topping'
- 2 peaches
- 6 fresh ripe apricots
- 1 banana
- A pinch of cinnamon
- 2 inch piece of vanilla pod
- 1 1/2 tbsp psyllium husks (see ingredients notes)
- 12 dried apricots finely chopped (reserve 2 for decoration)

1 Soak the dates in the orange juice for a few hours. When you are ready to use remove the dates from the orange juice and place in the food processor, reserving the juice for later.

2 Drain and rinse the almonds and pecans and add to the food processor with the dates. Cut open the vanilla pod and scoop out the tiny black seeds and place in the processor with the other ingredients. Process all the ingredients until they form a ball, adding some orange juice if required. Firmly press the mixture into an 8" pie dish.

3 To make the filling, peel the banana, pit the peaches and apricots and add to the food processor. Add the seeds from the vanilla pod and cinnamon and process until smooth.

4 Once the filling has been processed enough add the psyllium, immediately after this has blended in with the rest of the mixture stir in the chopped dried apricots.

5 Immediately spread the filling over the crust. Cut the remaining 2 apricots into slivers and decorate. Leave to set in the fridge for a few hours and serve.

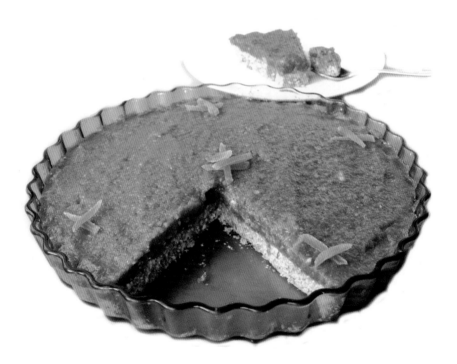

Orange & Fig 'Crema'

'Base'
- 2 cups walnuts soaked overnight in water
- 1/2 cup raisins soaked in orange juice overnight (1 orange)
- 1 tbsp raw carob powder

'Topping'
- 10 dried figs soaked in orange juice over night (1 orange)
- 6 fresh figs
- The zest of 1 orange
- 1 cup pine nuts

1 Drain and rinse the walnuts and place in the food processor, add the drained raisins (reserving the juice) and the carob. Process until the nuts and raisins stick together and form a ball.

2 Press the walnut mixture into a pie dish and set aside.

3 Wash the food processor and put the drained dried figs (reserving the juice), fresh figs and orange zest and process until smooth. Add the pine nuts and process again until all the pine nuts have been broken down and the mixture has taken on a creamy texture.

4 Smooth the topping over the walnut base and decorate with fresh fig quarters. Place in the fridge to thicken for a couple of hours before serving.

Halva

Sweet Sesame

- 1 cup sesame seeds
- 2 tbsp agave syrup
- 2 tbsp raw tahini

* Add any combination or one of the following:

- 2 tbsp chopped nuts (pistachios, cashews, pine nuts etc)
- 2 tbsp soaked raisins
- 1 tbsp carob powder

Grind the sesame seeds as finely as possible, place them in a bowl and add the tahini and agave syrup, mix thoroughly until there is an even consistency, and add the flavour of your choice. Press into a mould or form into a loaf shape and chill.

Cinnamon Biscuits

* Makes approximately 15 biscuits
- 2 cups pecans soaked overnight
- 1/2 cup flaxseeds ground
- 1/2 cup agave syrup
- 1/2 cup sultanas soaked
- 3 tbsp cinnamon
- 1/2 tsp salt
- The seeds from an inch of vanilla pod
- 1 tbsp sesame seeds for decoration

1 Drain and rinse the pecans and put in the food processor with the agave syrup, cinnamon and salt. Process until the pecans have all been ground down, and the mixture begins to form a ball.

2 Add to a bowl with the ground flax seeds and vanilla seeds and massage together with your hands.

3 Taking small amounts of the mixture in the hand mould into finger shaped biscuits. Lay onto a dehydrator tray and sprinkle with sesame seeds. Dehydrate at 118°F for about 3 hours and then at 100°F for approximately 2 hours.

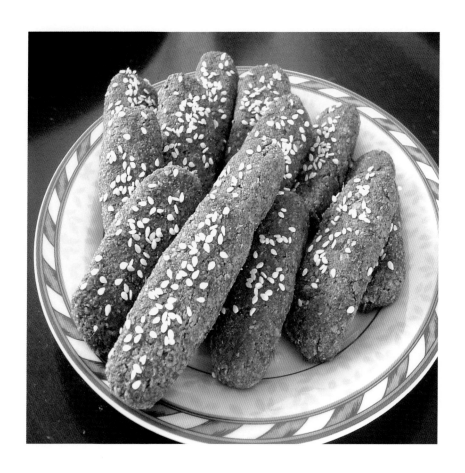

Plum Pudding

'Base'
- 1 1/2 cups almonds soaked
- 1 1/2 cups raisins soaked overnight
- 2 tbsp carob powder

'Topping'
- 4 cups pitted chopped plums
- 2 cups dried dates, pitted
- 3 bananas
- 1 tbsp psyllium husks (see ingredients notes)

1 Grind the almonds in the food processor, remove and then process the raisins.

2 Add the almonds and carob powder to the raisins and process until the ingredients form a smooth ball together. You may need to add a drop or two of water to make it rotate and stick better. Evenly press the mixture into an 8" pie dish and set aside.

3 Blend or process the dates and bananas until smooth. Add the psyllium and immediately after this has blended in with the rest of the mixture add the chopped plums and pulsate so that the plums are not completely dissolved and some remain partially chopped.

4 Immediately transfer the filling into the crust. Leave to set in the fridge for a few hours before serving.

" "The Doctor of the future will no longer treat the human frame with drugs, but rather will cure and prevent disease with nutrition"."

Thomas Edison (1870)

Raw fresh juices have a huge health affirming effect on the body and mind. Drinking a fresh juice delivers nutrients, vitamins, minerals, enzymes and countless other phytonutrients (nutrients derived from plants) to the body in an easily absorbed form.

The fruits and vegetables have already been broken down therefore the body does not need to work so hard to digest and is able to absorb the nutrients almost immediately into the body.

DRINKS

Juices
Melon & Lettuce
Peach & Cucumber
Orange & Spinach
Celery & Grape

Smoothies
Kiwi & Nectarine
Apricot & Orange
Frappe

Juices

Melon & Lettuce

- 1 slice water melon about 2.5 inches in width with skin
- 6 lettuce leaves (cos or romaine)

Put the melon through the juicer with the skin on followed by the lettuce leaves.

Peach & Cucumber

- 1/2 medium cucumber
- 3 stalks with leaves of fresh mint
- 2-3 peaches depending on how sweet they are

Put all the ingredients through the juicer making a point not to leave the mint until last.

Orange & Spinach

- 2 oranges
- 2 handfuls spinach

Juice the oranges using a citrus juicer. Put the spinach through a standard juicer. Mix the two juices together and serve.

Celery & Grape

- 750g red grapes
- 3 sticks celery

Put all the ingredients in the food processor including the pips of the grapes and blend until it becomes liquid. Strain the liquid using a nut milk bag and serve

* All serve 2

Smoothies

Kiwi & Nectarine

- 2 kiwis peeled
- 4 nectarines stoned
- 1 banana peeled

Put all the ingredients in the blender and blend until all the fruit has been liquidised.

Apricot & Orange

- 8 ripe apricots
- 2 oranges juiced using a citrus juicer
- 2 tbsp pine nuts

Put all the ingredients in the blender and blend until all the fruit has been liquidised.

'Frappe'

- $1/2$ honeydew melon
- 4 tsp raw agave syrup
- $1/2$ tsp carob powder
- 1 tsp tahini
- $1/8$ tsp cinnamon

Peel slice and cut the melon, place in the blender with the remaining ingredients and blend until the melon has dissolved.
Serve in a tall glass with ice.

* All serve 2

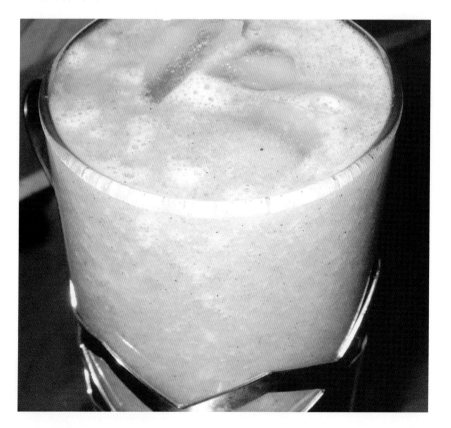

MEZE MENU IDEAS

A great delight of Greek life is the Meze, a civilized custom of sharing many small platters of food. The Meze table is where an appealing array of tempting, bite-sized titbits are laid out and shared amongst friends.

The skill of composing a successful meze table lies in the balance of ingredients and the essence of the meze experience is the surprise and pleasure of sampling a variety of intense contrasting flavours and textures in tiny mouthfuls. Platters of food such as *olives*, crunchy vegetables (fresh and preserved), *dips* and pulses appeal to the taste buds opening the appetite to the slightly heavier dishes such as 'meat'balls, *dolmadakia* and *stuffed tomatoes* and ending with a platter of fresh fruit.

Below I have listed some of the recipes from this book that would be suitable for a meze table, in the order that they might be served in a restaurant. However, be as bold as you like; invent new ideas by mixing and matching components from one or more recipes or move things around.

Olive spread
Houmus
Tzatziki
Meze Vegetables

Olives
'Sautéed' Mushrooms
Marinated Beetroot
Melitzanosalata

Dolmadakia
Stuffed tomatoes

Yiahni
Rouvithi

Village salad
Pilafi
'Rice'

Sheftalies
Koftedes

A platter of fresh chopped fruit or vegetables to end

SAMPLE MENUS

Below are some suggestions for 3 course menus; however, you can adjust them, add or remove dishes to suit your personal taste.

Menu 1
Marinated Olives
Barayemista served with *Melitzanosalata*
Apricot & Orange Smoothie

Menu 2
Tzatziki and celery sticks
Koftedes served with *'Sautéed' Mushrooms*
Orange & Fig Crema

Menu 3
Marinated Beetroot
Sheftalies served with *Pilafi*
Peach & Apricot Pie

Menu 4
Houmus and carrot batons
Moussaka served with *Village Salad*
Melomacarouna
Frappe

RAW RESOURCES

Suppliers of uncommon raw foods and equipment

The Fresh Network
www.fresh-network.com
PO Box 71
Ely
CB7 4GU
UK
Tel: +44 (0) 870 800 7070
Fax: +44 (0) 870 800 7071
E-mail: info@fresh-network.com

Rawcreation Ltd
www.rawcreation.com
Rawcreation Ltd
PO Box 223
Belton
Great Yarmouth
NR31 9WX
Tel: +44 (0) 8700 113 119
E-mail: info@rawcreation.com

Nature's First Law
www.rawfood.com
PO Box 900202
San Diego, CA 92190, USA
Tel: +1 (619)596 7979
Tel Orders: +1 (800) 205 2350
Fax: +1 (619) 596 7997
Email: nature@rawfood.com

UK Juicers
www.ukjuicers.com
UK Juicers Limited
Unit 5 Harrier Court
Airfield Business Park
Elvington
YORK
YO41 4EA
United Kingdom
Tel: +44 (0)1904 757070
Fax :   +44 (0)1904 757071
Email: enquiries@ukjuicers.com

Other useful resources

Raw Chef Training

Vital Creations
www.rawchef.org
Tel: +1 888 276 7170
Email: info@rawchef.org

Digital Raw Radio
Raw Vegan Radio
www.Rawveganradio.com

Magazines

Funky Raw
www.funkyraw.com
Tel: +44 (0) 207 193 6331
E-mail: rob@funkyraw.com
         holly@rawcuisine.co.uk

Living Nutrition
www.livingnutrition.com
P.O. Box 256
Sebastopol
CA 95473
Tel: +1 (707) 829-0362

Just Eat and Apple
www.justeatanapple.com
Living Foods Technology
P.O. Box 6783
Scarborough, ME 04070
USA
Email: info@justeatanapple.com

Lifescape Magazine
www.lifescapemag.co.uk
219 Canalot Studios
222 Kensal Road
London W10 5BN
Tel: +44 (0) 208 960 9494

Fresh Magazine
(Details above)

CREDITS

Thank you to everyone who offered me food suggestions and ideas and to those already pioneering raw foodists who have made me see that there are no limits.
Without the current availability of books, websites and lectures etc I would not have been able to produce this work, therefore I thank everybody for making the information readily available to myself and the rest of the world.

BIBLIOGRAPHY

Brian R. Clement with Theresa Foy Digeronimo (1998): Living Foods for Optimum Health. Prima Publishing

Chad Sarno (2002): Vital Creations, An Organic Life Experience.

David Wolfe (2003): Eating for Beauty. Maul Brothers Publishing

Eric Schlosser (2001): Fast Food Nation. The Penguin Press

Gabriel Cousens (2003): Rainbow Green Live-Food Cuisine. North Atlantic Books

Harvey & Marilyn Diamond (2004): Fit for Life. Bantam

John Robbins (1998): Diet for a New America. H J Kramer

Kate Wood (2002): Eat Smart Eat Raw. Grub Street

Leslie Kenton (2001): The New Raw Energy. Vermilion

Mike Nash (2002): Raw Perfection. Raw Perfection

Paul Nisson (2001): The Raw Life. 343 Publishing Company

Robert O. Young & Shelley R. Young (2000): Sick and Tired. Woodland Publishing

Shazzie (2003): Detox your World. Rawcreation Limited

Susan Miller & Karen Knowler (2000): Feel Good Food. The Women's Press Ltd

Suzanne Alex Ferrara (2003): The Raw Food Primer. Council Oak Books

RECIPE INDEX